THE WINI

EPILE

&

SEIZURE

DIET COOKBOOK

Cook Smart, Eat Well with The ESSENTIAL Dietary Guide to Track Seizures, Identify Triggers, Brain Trauma, Idiopathic Seizures and Epilepsy

Jessica Brown

COPYRIGHT PAGE

Table of Contents

Introduction

Epilepsy is defined as two or more unprovoked seizures, although the diagnosis may become apparent after initial presentation of a single seizure where the risk for recurrence is high. Some seizures never present after a single seizure, such as those persons with epilepsy (PWE) and absence or myoclonic seizures. Epilepsy is the world's most common serious neurologic disorder, affecting approximately 50 million individuals worldwide, with 25% unable to be controlled despite treatment. Within North America, more than 2.5 million persons have recurrent unprovoked seizures with an incidence of 50 persons per 100,000 per year or a prevalence of 5-10/1000 people. Epilepsy is a chronic disorder of the cerebral cortex with various etiologies characterized by recurrent seizures due to an excessive paroxysmal discharge of cortical neurons, associated with a variety of semiologic manifestations. A single seizure and acute symptomatic seizures during an acute illness or acute injury therefore are not synonymous with epilepsy. Epilepsy is thus defined as a disorder in which repeated seizures arise spontaneously in the same patient. Having more than two seizures carries a high risk of ongoing seizures, and though some patients with single seizures have a high risk, epilepsy is arguably evident when two unprovoked seizures occur. For many people seizures represent not only a clinical disorder that requires medical care, but also a condition with an important stigmatizing social impact. Dating from ancient history, epileptic seizures have been linked to religion and have represented a "sacred disease." Today however, misperceptions about epileptic seizures have been perpetuated by the public perception of the "grand mal" seizure as the sine qua non for epilepsy, creating continued misconception. In the media and film industry, seizures have been portrayed as convulsions, with patients "foaming at the mouth" in The Andromeda Strain, exhibiting demonic possession in The Exorcist, and with psychiatric association in A Beautiful Mind to impart a negative connotation for PWE. For many people, seizures produce an even greater adverse reaction than other stigma provoking conditions, including psychiatric conditions and HIV. Still, there exists the misperception by many Americans that seizures are a form of mental illness or that they may be contagious. For PWE, recurrent seizures have a significant adverse effect upon the quality of the individual's lifestyle— impairing driving, employment, socialization, and cognition—that extends far beyond the independent impact of the medical treatment.

The first time is always scary.

Seizures aren't the same for everyone: they are manifested differently for each person. We think of seizures as violent jerking or stiffening of the body with the victims suddenly finding themselves on the ground. Others, however, may experience different physical signs, including visual or hearing disturbances, abnormal electrical sensations or numbness, abruptly waking up, urinary discharge, and even staring blankly into space.

Seizures, no matter their appearances, can cause terrifying experiences and result in physical and psychological consequences for the victim.

The term epilepsy is used to identify individuals who have suffered two or more seizures.

If you or a loved one has been diagnosed with epilepsy, you are not alone. According to the Epilepsy Foundation, approximately 3.4 million Americans suffer from epilepsy. This disorder is far more common than most people realize, but it rarely gets the public attention it deserves.

Seizures and resultant epilepsy are often caused by head trauma. When seizures are caused by a head or brain injury, it is referred to as post-traumatic epilepsy. It is estimated that trauma causes 20% of symptomatic epilepsy. Seizures may have other causes, including neurological disorders such as a tumor6 or stroke. In approximately half of those diagnosed with epilepsy, however, the cause is unknown.

Epilepsy is generally not diagnosed until one experiences a second seizure, usually within a short time after the first. Given the complex and often mysterious nature of seizures, even the best medical professionals cannot identify epilepsy from just a single occurrence. Seizures can occur within moments, days, weeks, months, or even years following head trauma. Seizures occurring shortly after trauma increase the risk for developing further seizures.

Therefore, when one has a second seizure he or she is faced with a terrifying realization: this may be a permanent part of my life.

Yes, the first time is scary. The second time, however, represents the beginning of a pattern.

What Is Epilepsy?

Epilepsy is a neurological condition involving the brain that makes people more susceptible to having recurrent unprovoked seizures. It is one of the most common disorders of the nervous system and affects people of all ages, races and ethnic background. According to the CDC, almost 3 million Americans live with epilepsy and nearly 200,000 people in the U.S. develop this condition annually.

Anything that interrupts the normal connections between nerve cells in the brain can cause a seizure; this includes a high fever, low blood sugar, alcohol or drug withdrawal, or a brain concussion. Under these circumstances, anyone can have one or more seizures. However, when a person has two or more recurrent unprovoked seizures, he or she is considered to have epilepsy. There are many possible causes of epilepsy, including an imbalance of nerve-signaling chemicals called neurotransmitters, tumors, strokes, and brain damage from illness or injury, or some combination of these. In the majority of cases, there may be no detectable cause for epilepsy.

What Is a Seizure?

The brain is the center that controls and regulates all voluntary and involuntary responses in the body. It consists of nerve cells that normally communicate with each other through electrical activity.

A seizure occurs when part(s) of the brain receives a burst of abnormal electrical signals that temporarily interrupts normal electrical brain function.

What Are the Different Types of Seizures?

The type of seizure depends on which part and how much of the brain is affected and what happens during the seizure. The two broad categories of epileptic seizures are generalized seizures (absence, atonic, tonic-clonic, myoclonic) and partial (simple and complex) seizures. Within these categories, there are several different types of seizures in children, including:

Focal seizures. Focal seizures take place when abnormal electrical brain function occurs in one or more areas of one side of the brain. Focal seizures may also be called partial seizures. With focal seizures, particularly with complex focal seizures, the child may experience an aura before the seizure occurs. The most common aura involves feelings such as deja vu, impending doom, fear, or euphoria.

Visual changes, hearing abnormalities, or changes in the sense of smell can also be auras. Two types of partial seizures include:

Simple focal seizures. The child may show different symptoms depending upon which area of the brain is involved. If the abnormal electrical brain function is in the occipital lobe (the back part of the brain that is involved with vision), the child's sight may be altered. However, more commonly, a child's muscles are affected. The seizure activity is limited to an isolated muscle group, such as fingers or to larger muscles in the arms and legs. Consciousness is not lost in this type of seizure. The child may also experience sweating, nausea, or become pale.

Complex focal seizures. This type of seizure commonly occurs in the temporal lobe of the brain, the area of the brain that controls emotion and memory function. This seizure usually lasts one to two minutes. Consciousness is usually lost during these seizures. Losing consciousness may not mean that a child passes out--sometimes, a child stops being aware of what's going on around him or her. The child may look awake but have a variety of behaviors. These behaviors may range from gagging, lip smacking, running, screaming, crying, and/or laughing. When the child regains consciousness, he or she may complain of being tired or sleepy after the seizure. This is called the postictal period.

Generalized seizures. Generalized seizures involve both sides of the brain. There is loss of consciousness and a postictal state after the seizure occurs. Types of generalized seizures include the following:

Absence seizures (also called petit mal seizures). These seizures are characterized by a brief altered state of consciousness and staring episodes. Typically the child's posture is maintained during the seizure. The mouth or face may move or the eyes may blink. The seizure usually lasts no longer than 30 seconds. When the seizure is over, the child may not recall what just occurred and may go on with his/her activities, acting as though nothing happened. These seizures may occur several times a day. This type of seizure is sometimes mistaken for a learning problem or behavioral problem. Absence seizures almost always start between ages 4 to 12 years.

Atonic (also called drop attacks). With atonic seizures, there is a sudden loss of muscle tone and the child may fall from a standing position or suddenly drop his/her head. During the seizure, the child is limp and unresponsive.

Generalized tonic-clonic seizures (also called grand mal seizures). The classic form of this kind of seizure, which may not occur in every case, is characterized by five distinct phases. The body, arms, and legs will flex (contract), extend (straighten out), tremor (shake), a clonic period (contraction and relaxation of the muscles), followed by the postictal period. Not all of these phases may be seen with every one of this type of seizure. During the postictal period, the child may be sleepy, have problems with vision or speech, and may have a bad headache, fatigue, or body aches.

Myoclonic seizures. This type of seizure refers to quick movements or sudden jerking of a group of muscles. These seizures tend to occur in clusters, meaning that they may occur several times a day, or for several days in a row.

Infantile spasms. This rare type of seizure disorder occurs in infants from before six months of age. There is a high occurrence rate of this seizure when the child is awakening, or when they are trying to go to sleep. The infant usually has brief periods of movement of the neck, trunk, or legs that lasts for a few seconds. Infants may have hundreds of these seizures a day. This can be a serious problem, and can have long-term complications.

Febrile seizures. This type of seizure is associated with fever and is not epilepsy, although a fever may trigger a seizure in a child who has epilepsy. These seizures are more commonly seen in children between 6 months and 5 years of age and there may be a family history of this type of seizure. Febrile seizures that last less than 15 minutes are called "simple," and typically do not have long-term neurological effects. Seizures lasting more than 15 minutes are called "complex" and there may be long-term neurological changes in the child.

What Are the Symptoms of a Seizure?

The child may have varying degrees of symptoms depending on the type of seizure. The following are general symptoms of a seizure or warning signs that your child may be experiencing seizures. Symptoms or warning signs may include:

• Staring
• Jerking movements of the arms and legs
• Stiffening of the body
• Loss of consciousness
• Breathing problems or breathing stops
• Loss of bowel or bladder control
• Falling suddenly for no apparent reason, especially when associated with loss of consciousness
• Not responding to noise or words for brief periods
• Appearing confused or in a haze

• Nodding the head rhythmically, when associated with loss of awareness or even loss of consciousness
• Periods of rapid eye blinking and staring

During the seizure, the child's lips may become bluish and breathing may not be normal. The movements are often followed by a period of sleep or disorientation.

The symptoms of a seizure may resemble other problems or medical conditions. Always consult your child's doctor for a diagnosis.

What Causes a Seizure?

A child may experience one or many different types of seizures. While the exact cause of the seizure may not be known, the more common seizures are caused by the following:

In newborns and infants:

- Birth trauma
- Congenital (present at birth) problems
- Fever/infection
- Metabolic or chemical imbalances in the body

In children, adolescents, and young adults:

- Alcohol or drugs
- Trauma to the head or brain injury
- Infection

• Congenital conditions
• Genetic factors
• Unknown reasons

Other possible causes of seizures may include:

• Brain tumor
• Neurological problems
• Drug withdrawal
• Medications
• Use of illicit drugs

How Are Seizures Diagnosed?

The full extent of the seizure may not be completely understood immediately after onset of symptoms, but may be revealed with a comprehensive medical evaluation and diagnostic testing. The diagnosis of a seizure is made with a physical examination and diagnostic tests. During the examination, the physician obtains a complete medical history of the child and family and asks when the seizures occurred. Seizures may be due to neurological problems and require further medical follow up.

Diagnostic tests may include:

Blood tests

Electroencephalogram (EEG) - a procedure that records the brain's continuous, electrical activity by means of electrodes attached to the scalp.

Magnetic resonance imaging (MRI) - a diagnostic procedure that uses a combination of large magnets, radiofrequencies, and a computer to produce detailed images of organs and structures within the body.

Computed tomography scan (Also called a CT or CAT scan.) - a diagnostic imaging procedure that uses a combination of X-rays and computer technology to produce horizontal, or axial, images (often called slices) of the body. A CT scan shows detailed images of any part of the body, including the bones, muscles, fat, and organs. CT scans are more detailed than general X-rays.

Lumbar puncture (spinal tap) - a special needle is placed into the lower back, into the spinal canal. This is the area around the spinal cord. The pressure in the spinal canal and brain can then be measured. A small amount of cerebral spinal fluid (CSF) can be removed and sent for testing to determine if there is an infection or other problems. CSF is the fluid that bathes your child's brain and spinal cord.

How Are Seizures Treated?

- Specific treatment for a seizure will be determined by your child's doctor based on:
-
- • Your child's age, overall health, and medical history
- • Extent of the condition
- • Type of seizure
- • Your child's tolerance for specific medications, procedures, or therapies
- • Expectations for the course of the condition
- • Your opinion or preference
-
- The goal of seizure management is to control, stop, or decrease the frequency of the seizures without interfering with the child's normal growth and development. The major goals of seizure management include the

following: Proper identification of the type of seizure

- • Using medication specific to the type of seizure
- • Using the least amount of medication to achieve adequate control
- • Maintaining good medicating levels

Treatment may include:

Medications

There are many types of medications used to treat seizures and epilepsy. Medications are selected based on the type of seizure, age of the child, side effects, the cost of the medication, and the adherence with the use of the medication.

Medications used at home are usually taken by mouth (as capsules, tablets, sprinkles, or syrup), but some can be given rectally (into the child's rectum). If the child is in the hospital with seizures, medication by injection or intravenous (IV) may be used.

It is important to give your child his/her medication on time and as prescribed by your child's physician. Different people use up the medication in their body differently, so adjustments (schedule and dosage) may need to be made for good control of seizures.

All medications can have side effects, although some children may not experience side effects. Discuss your child's medication side effects with his/her physician.

While your child is taking medications, different tests may be done to monitor the effectiveness of the medication. These tests may include the following:

Blood work - frequent blood draws testing is usually required to check the level of the medication in the body. Based on this level, the physician may increase or decrease the dose of the medication to achieve the desired level. This level is called the "therapeutic level" and is where the medication works most efficiently. Blood work may also be done to monitor the affects of medications on body organs.

Urine tests - these tests are performed to see how the child's body is responding to the medication.

Electroencephalogram (EEG) - a procedure that records the brain's continuous, electrical activity by means of electrodes attached to the scalp. This test is done to monitor how the medication is helping the electrical problems in the brain.

Ketogenic diet - Certain children who are having problems with medications, or whose seizures are not being well controlled, may be placed on a special diet called the ketogenic diet. This type of diet is low in carbohydrates and high in protein and fat.

The 3 Stages of a Seizure

No matter what the cause or trigger, individuals experiencing a seizure often go through several distinct stages. These stages are named: auras, ictal, and postictal.30

Stage 1: Aural Stage

The aura stage is the beginning of the seizure and often only lasts for seconds or minutes. Not all seizures start with a distinct aura stage, but many do. The symptoms in the aura stage are usually only noticeable by the patient themselves and are not visible to the outside observer.

People experiencing an aura stage often describe abnormal feelings or sensations, such as déjà vu, out-of-body experiences, or "phantom" sounds, tastes, or smells. Aura stages can be accompanied by physical sensations such as dizziness, nausea, headaches, numbness, or lightheadedness. People in the aura stage may experience heightened emotions, such as fear and panic.

Some seizures stop after the aura stage and leave the person aware and able to respond. Other seizures may proceed to other stages.

Stage 2: Ictal Stage

The ictal stage is the seizure itself.

When people think of a seizure, they are typically referring to the ictal stage. If the aura stage is the beginning of the seizure, this is the middle. Intense electrical charges are emitted in the brain. This stage is the actual seizure: the electrical storm is unleashed from your brain throughout your body.

Ictal stage symptoms are not just the tremors or jerking motions that most people associate with someone having a seizure. They can include sensory and cognitive changes similar to the aura stage.

The physical symptoms also vary widely from individual to individual. Some people "blackout," while others retain consciousness. Even if someone in the ictal stage is conscious, he/she may not be responsive. The seizure can cause someone to slur his or her speech, make only noises, or lose the ability to vocalize completely.

In contrast to the typical perception of a seizure, many people in the ictal stage stop moving. Their muscles may lock up so their bodies tense and stiffen like a board. They may lose control of neck and head muscles, resulting in their heads slumping forward.

Other common physical signs of a seizure can include drooling, repeated eye movements, sweating, dilated pupils, increased heart rate, and loss of urinary or bowel control.

Stage 3: Postictal Stage

The postictal stage is the recovery phase, after the seizure occurs.

It is when the brain and body recover from the seizure. Recovery looks different for everyone: some people recover immediately and can continue to perform regular tasks, while others may take minutes or even hours to feel like their usual selves. The average postictal stage lasts for 5-30 minutes.

Many people with epilepsy report feeling disoriented during the period immediately after the seizure. People may remember nothing about the seizure or may have a distorted memory of the event, further contributing to this sense of disorientation.

Another common sensation is physical exhaustion. The post-seizure exhaustion may last for several days.

Types of Epileptic Seizures

Seizures have been categorized and described in many ways. A group of the world's leading epilepsy professionals, the International League Against Epilepsy (ILAE), introduced a new process for classification in March 2017 to equip professionals with more accurate means of identifying types of seizures and prescribing the most appropriate treatments.

One core element of this improved classification process is seizures are defined and categorized by where they start in the brain.

Seizures that start in one area of the brain, are called focal seizures. Seizures that start in both sides of the brain, are called generalized seizures.

Some seizures, begin as a focal seizure and then progress to generalized seizures.
A secondary component of the updated classification identifies whether a person's awareness is affected during a focal seizure. This does not apply to generalized seizures, in which an individual's awareness will be affected.

The third element of the updated classification structure is whether the person displays motor symptoms. Motor symptoms include what many commonly think of as a seizure: jerking, twitching, or stiffening movements of a body part. Non-motor symptoms include the less visible bodily changes such as changes in sensations, emotions, thoughts, and experiences.

The ketogenic diet is sometimes offered to those children who continue to have seizures while on seizure medication. When the medications do not work, a ketogenic diet may be considered. No one knows exactly how the diet works, but some children do become seizure-free when put on the diet. However, the diet does not work for everyone.

What Does the Diet Consist of?

The ketogenic diet is very high in fat (about 90 percent of the calories come from fat). Protein is given in amounts to help promote growth. A very small amount of carbohydrate is included in the diet. This very high- fat, low- carbohydrate diet causes the body to make ketones. Ketones are made by the body from the breakdown of fat. They are made for energy when the body does not get enough carbohydrates for energy. If your child eats too many carbohydrates, then his/her body may not make ketones. The presence of ketones is important to the success of the diet.

High-fat foods:

- Butter
- Heavy cream
- Oil
- Mayonnaise
- Cream cheese
- Bacon
- Cheese

High-carbohydrate foods:

- Fruit and fruit juice

- Breads and cereals
- Vegetables (corn, peas, and potatoes)
- Beans
- Milk
- Soda
- Snack foods (chips, snack cakes, crackers)
- Sweets

Your child's doctor will determine if this diet is right for your child. When the ketogenic diet is started, your child will be admitted to the hospital. It may take four to five days in the hospital to get the diet started and for you to learn how to plan the diet.

While in the hospital, your child may not be able to eat for one to two days until ketones are measured in the urine. Once ketones are present in the urine, special high-fat, low-carbohydrate shakes may be started. These are sometimes called "keto shakes."

After several meals of keto shakes, your child will be started on solid foods.

You may also be taught how to check your child's urine for ketones. The dietitian will help determine how much fat, protein, and carbohydrate your child is allowed to have, usually divided into three meals a day. The ketogenic diet can by very challenging to prepare and requires that all foods be weighed using a food scale. The ketogenic diet is not nutritionally balanced, therefore, vitamin and mineral supplements are needed.

Some medications and other products, such as toothpaste and mouthwash, contain carbohydrates. It is important to avoid these products if your child is on the ketogenic diet. Your child may not make ketones in their urine if too many carbohydrates are included in the diet. Your child's doctor and dietitian can give you a list of medications, and other products, that are free of carbohydrates.

How Long Is the Diet Used?

Children usually stay on the diet for two years. The diet is slowly changed back to a regular diet.

Sample Ketogenic Meal

- 60g heavy cream
- 21 g strawberries
- 53 g eggs
- 10 g cheddar cheese
- 10 g bacon
- 21 g butter

Sample Ketogenic Shake

- 500 g Ross Carbohydrate-free Formula (concentrate)
- 270 g heavy cream
- 13 g Egg Beaters

Additional Treatment Options:

Vagus nerve stimulation (VNS): Some children, whose seizures are not being well-controlled with seizure medications, may benefit from a procedure called vagus nerve stimulation (VNS). VNS is currently most commonly used for children over the age of 12 who have partial seizures that are not controlled by other methods.

VNS attempts to control seizures by sending small pulses of energy to the brain from the vagus nerve, which is a large nerve in the neck. This is done by surgically placing a small battery into the chest wall. Small wires are then attached to the battery and placed under the skin and around the vagus nerve. The battery is then programmed to send energy impulses every few minutes to the brain. When the child feels a seizure coming on, he/she may activate the impulses by holding a small magnet over the battery. In many people, this will help to stop the seizure.

There are some side of the effects that may occur with the use of VNS. These may include, but are not limited to, the following:

- Hoarseness
- Pain or discomfort in the throat
- Change in voice

Surgery. Another treatment option for seizures is surgery. Surgery may be considered in a child who:

• Has seizures that are unable to be controlled with medications.

• Has seizures that always start in one area of the brain.

• Has a seizure in a part of the brain that can be removed without disrupting important behaviors such as speech, memory, or vision.

Surgery for epilepsy and seizures is a very complicated surgery performed by a specialized surgical team. The operation may remove the part of the brain where the seizures are occurring, or, sometimes, the surgery helps to stop the spread of the bad electrical currents through the brain.

A child may be awake during the surgery. The brain itself does not feel pain. With the child awake and able to follow commands, the surgeons are better able to make sure that important areas of the brain are not damaged.

Dorene's Low Carb Almond Vanilla Pancakes

Please note that in different parts of the world different brands have more or less carbs. It is important to read the labels carefully when you shop for food. If you have difficulty locating low carb supplies, please visit our low carb supplier page for some items that can be ordered online.

Ingredients

5 Tbsp. almond flour you could also use other nut flours or even soy flour

1 1/2-2 tsp. flax meal this helps hold these together

1 Tbsp. sour cream

3 Tbsp. water

1 egg

1/2 tsp. baking powder

1/8 tsp sea salt

8 drops of liquid stevia

1/4 tsp. pure vanilla extract no sweeteners in it like Simply Organic

2 Tbsp. melted coconut oil

Instructions

Mix all the ingredients together and let sit a couple of minutes. If the consistency is too thick for your personal taste, you can add a bit more liquid (unsweetened almond milk, heavy whipping cream, or water).

Gina's Low Carb Blueberry Topping

Please note that in different parts of the world, different brands of available food have more carbs than other brands. It is important to read the labels carefully where you shop for food. If you have difficulty locating low carb supplies, please visit our low carb supplier page for some items that can be mail ordered.

Ingredients

Frozen blueberries

Vanilla crème liquid stevia

Alternative: a sprinkle of stevia powder and a tsp of vanilla

Instructions

Microwave frozen blueberries until hot or heat in a pan

Stir in drops if stevia to taste

The hot blueberries form a nice liquid syrup that's perfect to top buttered almond flour pancakes. This can also be used as a dessert dish or topping.

Dorene's Low Carb Hot Chocolate

Please note that in different parts of the world, different brands of available food have more carbs than other brands. It is important to read the labels carefully where you shop for food. If you have difficulty locating low carb supplies, please visit our low carb supplier page for some items that can be mail ordered.

Ingredients

¼ Cup heavy whipping cream

1 cup unsweetened almond milk this only has 2 grams carb per cup- it's Diamond brand

¾ cup water

1-2 tsp oil can be coconut or EVOO or melted butter to mix with cocoa powder

1 tbsp cocoa powder

Sweetener to taste we like 20 drops of stevia and 20 drops of Sweet 10

Dash of sea salt

Instructions

In a small pan heat the oil or butter until melted

Mix or whisk in the cocoa powder

Add the cream, milk, water, sweetener and salt and mix well

Simmer until it's heated through and give it a final whisk to make sure there is no "skin" on it

Pour into two cups

Mike's Low Carb Cheese Pizza

Please note that in different parts of the world different brands have more or less carbs. It is important to read the labels carefully when you shop for food. If you have difficulty locating low carb supplies, please visit our low carb supplier page for some items that can be ordered online.

Ingredients

½ cup cream cheese softened

2 eggs

¼ cup parmesan cheese grated

¼ teaspoon oregano or Italian seasoning

¼ teaspoon garlic powder

1 cup Italian cheese blend or mozzarella cheese shredded

¼ cup pizza sauce

½ cup mozzarella cheese shredded

Toppings: pepperoni ham, sausage, mushrooms, green peppers, bacon, ground beef, etc. Dash of garlic powder and some Italian seasoning

Instructions

In a medium bowl, whisk cream cheese until smooth and creamy

Whisk in eggs until mixture is well-blended and smooth

Add the grated parmesan and seasonings

Stir in 1 cup of mozzarella until completely mixed

Spread the mixture evenly onto a well-greased 9 x 13″ baking dish or large round pizza pan. We suggest lining the pan or dish with greased wax paper or a baking sheet

Bake at 375 for 20-25 minutes or until evenly browned, but not too dark

Let cool completely, then take a metal spatula and carefully pry up the edges to loosen from pan. Ease the spatula under the whole crust to loosen. Don't remove the crust from the pan, this makes it easier to remove the finished pizza

Spread the crust with pizza sauce, then cheese and toppings of your choice.

Lightly sprinkle with seasonings

Bake at 375 for 15-20 minutes or until cheese is bubbling

Let stand a few minutes before cutting

Low Carb Cauliflower Pizza

Please note that in different parts of the world, different brands of available food have more carbs than other brands. It is important to read the labels carefully where you shop for food. If you have difficulty locating low carb supplies, please visit our low carb supplier page for some items that can be mail ordered.

Ingredients

250 g/8.82 oz Cauliflower

30 g/1.06 oz grated Parmesan cheese

15 g/ 0.53 oz Cream Cheese

1 Egg

2 Tbsp low carb pizza sauce

50 g/1.76 oz grated cheese

Instructions

Seperate the cauliflower florets from the stems

Using a food processor wiz up the florets until fine but not mashed

Cook the cauliflower in a dry pan on medium heat for 5-6 minutes

Using a cloth or tea towel squeeze out all the liquid remaining in the cauliflower

Mix together the cream cheese, grated parmesan cheese, 1 egg, salt and pepper in a bowl. Add the cauliflower and mix together

Line a baking tray with parchment paper. Spoon your cauliflower mixture onto the tray and shape into a round base with your hands

Bake for 20 minutes in the oven at 374 Fahrenheit / 190 Celsius

Once cooked flip over and add your sauce, cheese and toppings

Return to the oven to bake until the cheese is melted

Low Carb Pizza Sauce

Please note that in different parts of the world, different brands of available food have more carbs than other brands. It is important to read the labels carefully where you shop for food. If you have difficulty locating low carb supplies, please visit our low carb supplier page for some items that can be mail ordered.

Ingredients

400 g/14.11 oz Tomatoes

50 g /1.76 oz Diced Red Onion

5 g/0.18 oz Chopped Garlic

2 tbsp Olive Oil

1 tbsp Butter

5 g/0.18 oz Fresh or Dried Oregano

A handful chopped basil

Instructions

Heat the Olive Oil in a saucepan

Add the chopped onion and a pinch of salt. Fry until the onion is translucent

Add the chopped garlic and cook until golden brown

Add the tomatoes and season with salt and pepper

Cover and cook for 10 minutes

Add the oregano and basil and cook for another 3 minutes

Add the butter at the end of cooking

Melanie's Low Carb Chocolate Chip Cookies

Please note that in different parts of the world different brands have more or less carbs. It is important to read the labels carefully when you shop for food. If you have difficulty locating low carb supplies, please visit our low carb supplier page for some items that can be ordered online.

Ingredients

1 cup almond flour

½ cup unsweetened coconut

1 tsp vanilla flavoring

½ cup CarbSense brand Mini-Carb semi-sweet chocolate chips

1 egg

Heavy cream to moisten mixture about ½ cup

Instructions

Preheat the oven to 350 degrees Fahrenheit/180 degrees celsius.

Mix all the ingredients together

Add enough cream to form a cookie dough consistency

Use a spoon to make small scoops of the dough and place them on a greased cookie sheet. Press down to desired thickness.

Bake for 17-20 minutes or until golden brown

Tammy's Low Carb Baked Ricotta Cakes

Please note that in different parts of the world different brands have more or less carbs. It is important to read the labels carefully when you shop for food. If you have difficulty locating low carb supplies, please visit our low carb supplier page for some items that can be ordered online.

Ingredients

1 cup ricotta cheese

2 egg whites beaten

⅙ cup sugar-free syrup

1 tsp vanilla

Instructions

Preheat oven to 350 degrees F.

Place the ricotta cheese in a bowl and break it up with a wooden spoon

Add the beaten egg whites, syrup and vanilla. Mix thoroughly until the mixture is smooth and well combined

Lightly grease four small ramekins or use a greased muffin tray

Bake for 20 minutes, or until the ricotta cakes have risen and are golden brown

Ingredients

4 ounces unsweetened chocolate can be any brand as long as it's unsweetened

1 and a half sticks of butter

1 ½ teaspoons Vanilla flavoring

1 cup Splenda or NoSugar

1 cup almond flour

3 eggs

Instructions

Melt chocolate and butter together in microwave or in a double boiler.

Blend well.

Add sugar and vanilla until well blended.

Mix in the eggs and then the almond flour.

Bake in a well-greased 8x8x2 baking pan at 350 fahrenheit or 180 degrees celsius for 30-35 minutes or until toothpick comes out almost clean.

Tammy's One Carb Peanut Butter Cookies

Please note that in different parts of the world, different brands of available food have more carbs than other brands. It is important to read the labels carefully where you shop for food. If you have difficulty locating low carb supplies, please visit our low carb supplier page for some items that can be mail ordered.

Ingredients

½ cup plus natural creamy peanut butter

¼ cup room temp butter

2 eggs

2/3 cup heavy whipping cream

½ tsp baking soda

¼ tsp sea salt

stevia to taste we use about 20 drops

Instructions

Mix all of the ingredients together. Make sure that the butter is soft enough to easily mix in.

Line a baking tray with a cookie sheet.

Spoon on tablespoons of mix, leaving room between cookies. The mix will be wet but should hold it's shape.

Bake at 375 degrees F. for 11 minutes or until done.

Keto Stuffed Cabbage

Ingredients

For the sauce:

1 (14-oz.) can diced tomatoes

1 tbsp. apple cider vinegar

1/2 tsp. red pepper flakes

1 tsp. onion powder

1 tsp. garlic powder

1 tsp. dried oregano

Kosher salt

Freshly ground black pepper

1/4 c. extra-virgin olive oil

For the cabbage rolls:

12 cabbage leaves

1 lb. ground beef

3/4 lb. ground pork

1 c. riced cauliflower

3 green onions, thinly sliced

1/4 c. chopped parsley, plus more for serving

Freshly ground black pepper

Directions

For the sauce:

Preheat oven to 375°. Puree tomatoes, apple cider vinegar, red pepper flakes, onion powder, garlic powder, and oregano in a blender; season with salt and pepper.

In a large deep skillet (or large pot) over medium heat, heat oil. Add pureed tomato sauce, bring to a simmer, then lower to medium-low and simmer for 20 minutes, until slightly thickened.

For the cabbage rolls:

In a large pot of boiling water, blanch cabbage leaves until tender and flexible, about 1 minute. Set aside.

Make filling: in a large bowl, combine ½ c. tomato sauce, ground meats, cauliflower rice, scallions, and parsley. Season with salt and pepper.

Spread a thin layer of sauce on the bottom of a large baking dish. Using a paring knife, cut out the hard triangular rib from each cabbage leaf. Place about ⅓ cup filling into one end of each leaf, then roll up, tucking in the sides as you roll. Place rolls seam side-down on top of sauce in baking dish. Spoon remaining sauce on top of cabbage rolls. Bake 45 minutes to 55 minutes, until the meat is cooked through and internal temperature reaches 150°" Garnish with more parsley before serving.

Keto Meatballs

Ingredients

For The Meatballs

1 lb. ground beef

1 clove garlic, minced

1/2 c. shredded mozzarella

1/4 c. freshly grated Parmesan, plus more for serving

2 tbsp. freshly chopped parsley

1 large egg, beaten

1 tsp. kosher salt

1/2 tsp. freshly ground black pepper

2 tbsp. extra-virgin olive oil

For The Sauce

1 medium onion, chopped

2 cloves garlic, minced

1 (28-oz.) can crushed tomatoes

1 tsp. dried oregano

Kosher salt

Freshly ground black pepper

Directions

In a large bowl combine beef, garlic, mozzarella, Parmesan, parsley, egg, salt, and pepper. Form into 16 meatballs.

In a large skillet over medium heat, heat oil. Add meatballs and cook, turning occasionally, until golden on all sides, about 10 minutes. Remove from skillet and place on a paper towel-lined plate.

To the same skillet, add onion and cook until soft, 5 minutes. Add garlic and cook until fragrant, 1 minute more. Add tomatoes and oregano and season with salt and pepper.

Add meatballs back to skillet, cover and simmer until sauce has thickened, 15 minutes. Garnish with Parmesan before serving.

Keto Broccoli Salad

Ingredients

For The Salad

Kosher salt

3 heads broccoli, cut into bite-size pieces

1/2 c. Cheddar, shredded

1/4 red onion, thinly sliced

1/4 c. toasted sliced almonds

3 slices bacon, cooked and crumbled

2 tbsp. freshly chopped chives

For The Dressing

2/3 c. mayonnaise

3 tbsp. apple cider vinegar

1 tbsp. dijon mustard

Kosher salt

Freshly ground black pepper

Directions

In a medium pot or saucepan, bring 6 cups of salted water to a boil. While waiting for the water to boil, prepare a large bowl with ice water.

Add broccoli florets to the boiling water and cook until tender, 1 minute. Remove with a slotted spoon and immediately place in the prepared bowl of ice water. When cool, spin the broccoli in a salad spinner. You will need to spin it at least twice.

In a medium bowl, whisk to combine dressing ingredients. Season to taste with salt and pepper.

Combine all salad ingredients in a large bowl and pour over dressing. Toss until ingredients are combined and fully coated in dressing. Refrigerate until ready to serve.

Baked Pork Chops

Ingredients

4 pork loin chops

kosher salt

Freshly ground black pepper

1 tbsp. freshly minced rosemary

2 cloves garlic, minced

1/2 c. (1 stick) butter, melted

1 tbsp. extra-virgin olive oil

Directions

Preheat oven to 375°. Season pork chops generously with salt and pepper.

In a small bowl mix together butter, rosemary, and garlic. Set aside.

In an oven safe skillet over medium-high heat, heat olive oil then add pork chops. Sear until golden, 4 minutes, flip and cook 4 minutes more. Brush pork chops generously with garlic butter.

Place skillet in oven and cook until cooked through (145° for medium), 10-12 minutes. Serve with more garlic butter.

Cheesy Bacon Ranch Chicken

Ingredients

4 slices thick-cut bacon

4 boneless skinless chicken breasts (about 1 3/4 lbs.)

Kosher salt

Freshly ground black pepper

2 tsp. ranch seasoning

1 1/2 c. shredded mozzarella

Chopped chives, for garnish

Directions

In a large skillet over medium heat, cook bacon, flipping once, until crispy, about 8 minutes. Transfer to a paper towel lined plate. Drain all but 2 tablespoons of bacon fat from the skillet.

Season chicken with salt and pepper. Return skillet to medium-high heat, add chicken and cook until golden and just cooked through, about 6 minutes per side.

Reduce heat to medium and sprinkle chicken with ranch seasoning and top with mozzarella. Cover the skillet and cook, until cheese is melted and bubbly, about 5 minutes.

Crumble and sprinkle bacon and chives on top before serving.

Keto Taco Casserole

Ingredients

1 tbsp. extra-virgin olive oil

1/2 yellow onion, diced

2 lb. ground beef

2 tbsp. kosher salt

Freshly ground black pepper

2 tbsp. keto taco seasoning mix

1 jalapeño, seeded and minced, plus more sliced for garnish

6 large eggs, lightly beaten

2 c. shredded Mexican cheese

2 tbsp. freshly chopped parsley leaves

1 c. sour cream, for serving (optional)

Directions

Preheat oven to 350°. In a large skillet over medium heat, heat oil. Add onion and cook until slightly softened, 2 minutes.

Add ground beef and season with salt and pepper. Cook, breaking up meat with a wooden spoon, until no longer pink, 6 minutes. Sprinkle in taco seasoning and jalapeño and cook, stirring, until spices are lightly toasted, 1 minute. Drain and let cool slightly.

In a large mixing bowl, whisk eggs, then add in meat mixture. Spread mixture into an even layer in the bottom of a 2-quart baking dish. Sprinkle with cheese.

Bake until set, about 25 minutes.

Sprinkle with parsley and top each slice with a dollop of sour cream and jalapeño, if desired.

Keto Chicken Parmesan

Ingredients

4 boneless skinless chicken breasts

Kosher salt

Freshly ground black pepper

1 c. almond flour

3 large eggs, beaten

3 c. freshly grated Parmesan, plus more for serving

2 tsp. garlic powder

1 tsp. onion powder

2 tsp. dried oregano

Vegetable oil

3/4 c. low-carb sugar-free tomato sauce

1 1/2 c. shredded mozzarella

Fresh basil leaves, for topping

Directions

Preheat oven to 400°. Using a sharp knife, cut chicken breasts in half crosswise. Season chicken on both sides with salt and pepper.

Place eggs and almond flour in 2 separate shallow bowls. In a third shallow bowl, combine Parmesan, garlic powder, onion powder, and oregano. Season with salt and pepper.

Working with one at a time, dip chicken cutlets into almond flour, then eggs, and then Parmesan mixture, pressing to coat.

In a large skillet over medium heat, heat 2 tablespoons oil. Add chicken and cook until golden and cooked through, 2 to 3 minutes per side. Work in batches as necessary, adding more oil when needed.

Transfer fried cutlets to a 9"-x-13" baking dish, evenly spread tomato sauce on each cutlet and top with mozzarella.

Bake until cheese is melty, 10 to 12 minutes. If desired, broil until cheese is golden, 3 minutes.

Top with basil and more Parmesan before serving.

Bacon-Wrapped Keto Meatloaf

Ingredients

Cooking spray

1 tbsp. extra-virgin olive oil

1 medium onion, chopped

1 stalk celery, chopped

3 cloves garlic, minced

1 tsp. dried oregano

1 tsp. chili powder

2 lb. ground beef

1 c. shredded cheddar

1/2 c. almond flour

1/4 c. grated Parmesan

2 eggs

1 tbsp. low-sodium soy sauce

Kosher salt

Freshly ground black pepper

6 thin strips bacon

Directions

Preheat oven to 400°. Grease a medium baking dish with cooking spray. In a medium skillet over medium heat, heat oil. Add onion and celery and cook until soft, 5 minutes. Stir in garlic, oregano, and chili powder and cook until fragrant, 1 minute. Let mixture cool slightly.

In a large bowl, combine ground beef, vegetable mixture, cheese, almond flour, Parmesan, eggs, soy sauce, and season with salt and pepper. Shape into a large loaf in baking dish, then lay bacon slices on top.

Cook until bacon is crispy and beef is cooked through, about 1 hour. If bacon is cooking too quickly, cover dish with foil.

Delicious meat roll.

Ingredients:

700 g of any minced meat,

two slices of dried bread,

five chicken eggs, up to 400 g of champignons,

2 pcs. Bulbs, one carrot, some salt, cold water,

sunflower oil (or other).

We begin to cook:

Peeled washed mushrooms cut into medium pieces, chop the onions, carrots rub on the grater.

We admit in a frying pan with butter mushrooms, carrots and ½ of sliced onions, add salt to taste, stir and leave to stew. In the meantime, cook three eggs, cool and clean. Average sliced. Pieces of bread moisten with water, squeeze, let's go through the meat grinder along with the remaining onions. Add meat mince, 2 raw eggs and 2 tablespoons of cold water, salt, spices. We mix. Three quarters of the stuffing is distributed on a cellophane food film in the form of a rectangle with a layer of about 15 mm. Top with a layer of mushrooms with vegetables, not reaching the edges of minced meat approximately 15 mm. Over the mushrooms distribute chopped boiled eggs and wrap the structure with roll (it is convenient to do with wet hands). Carefully transfer the roll to the oiled baking tray (you can shift it with baking paper). If the cracks are formed

during the transfer, carefully lubricate them with deferred minced meat. We send it to a hot oven at a temperature of 180 ° C for about 60 minutes, until it is ready. Usually roll is served hot.
Garnish can be prepared with potatoes.

Ham and cheese salad.

We need:

green salad leaves,

cucumbers,

cherry tomatoes,

green onions,

ham,

cheese (brynza or mozzarella),

boiled eggs,

salt,

olive oil and lemon juice.

The number of ingredients is arbitrary - it still turns out delicious.

We start cooking:

all the ingredients are cut into medium pieces, poured with olive oil dressing with lemon juice. Add salt to taste. Simple, fast and delicious!

Meat stew.

Ingredients

Products: 0,5 kg of meat,

100 g of onion,

two carrots,

two stalks of celery,

garlic to taste,

4 tomatoes,

1 tbsp. L. Tomato paste,

salt,

seasoning,

vegetable oil,

greens.

Preparation:

Meat cut into pieces about one by two centimeters.

Stew it in vegetable oil until cooked.

Finely chop the onions, carrots, garlic and celery.

Add to the stew and continue to simmer for about 10 minutes.

Then add the tomato paste and finely chopped tomatoes (preferably without the skin), as well as salt and seasonings.

Add a little water and simmer on low heat. After the ragout is ready, sprinkle with herbs and serve it to the table. Bon Appetit!

No Knead Bread

Ingredients For No Knead Bread

2 c water

4 c all purpose flour

1 tsp bread machine yeast or quick yeast

1 3/4 tsp

salt

How To Make No Knead Bread

in large bowl mix dry ingredients then pour them into the 2 cups of water and mix. no need to overmix, just enough to moisten everything.

Put dough in large, greased, airtight container for 12 hours

On floured surface turn out dough, fold it into itself once or twice then dust with flour and cover with plastic wrap for 2 1/2 hours

Pre-heat oven to 500 degrees with your covered casserole dish or dutch oven inside. once the oven is hot, remove dish and carefully turn dough into it, cover and place in oven for half an hour.

Remove lid and bake another 10 minutes. remove from oven and turn bread out of dish. dont leave it in the baking dish as it will keep the bottom from becoming as crusty as it can be.
Allow bread to completely cool.

Soft burger buns

Combine the ingredients for brioche with a burger bun recipe to make a deliciously sweet, soft, light dough. It could also be shaped into hot dog rolls

Method

Put the milk, butter and 100ml water in a pan and gently heat until the butter is melted. Set aside to cool until just warm.
Tip the flour, sugar, yeast and 1 tsp salt into a large bowl and gradually work in the milk mixture, then the egg, until you have a smooth dough. Tip the dough onto a floured surface or into a stand mixer

fitted with a dough hook and knead until elastic and shiny. Divide into 12 (about 80g each) pieces and roll into tight balls. Transfer to baking trays lined with baking parchment, leaving plenty of space between them, and put in a warm place to prove for 30-45 mins.

Heat oven to 200C/180C fan/gas 6. Press the rolls down gently using your hands, then brush over some milk and scatter over the sesame seeds, if you like (or, dust with some flour). Bake for 10-12 mins until risen and lightly golden. Leave to cool completely, then serve. Make up to two days ahead and keep in an airtight container.

Low Carb Keto Sugar-Free Carrot Cake Recipe With Almond Flour

Ingredients

3/4 cup Besti Erythritol (or coconut sugar for paleo)

3/4 cup Butter (softened; use coconut or ghee for paleo or dairy-free)

1 tbsp Blackstrap molasses (optional)

1 tsp Vanilla extract

1/2 tsp Pineapple extract (optional)

4 large Eggs (preferably at room temperature)

2 1/2 cup Wholesome Yum Blanched Almond Flour

2 tsp Baking powder

2 tsp Cinnamon

1/2 tsp Sea salt

2 1/2 cup Carrots (grated, measured loosely packed after grating)

1 1/2 cup Pecans (chopped; divided into 1 cup and 1/2 cup)

2 full recipes Sugar-free cream cheese frosting (double the frosting recipe; for paleo or dairy-free, omit or use a coconut cream based frosting instead)

Instructions

Tap on the times in the instructions below to start a kitchen timer while you cook.

Preheat the oven to 350 degrees F (177 degrees C). Line two 9 in (23 cm) round cake pans with parchment paper. (Use springform pans if you have them.) Grease the bottom and sides.

In a large bowl, cream together the butter and erythritol, until fluffy. Beat in the molasses (if using), vanilla extract, and pineapple extract (if using). Beat in the eggs, one at a time. Set aside.

In another bowl, mix together the almond flour, baking powder, cinnamon, and sea salt. Stir the dry ingredients into the bowl with the wet ingredients. Stir in the grated carrots. Fold 1 cup (99 g) of the chopped pecans, reserving the remaining 1/2 cup (48.5 g).

Transfer the batter evenly among the two prepared baking pans. Bake for 30-35 minutes, until the top is spring-y.

Let the cakes cool in the pans for 10 minutes, then transfer to a wire rack to cool completely.

Meanwhile, make the sugar-free frosting according to the instructions here. (Double the recipe by entering "12" into the box for # of servings on that page.)

When the cake has cooled to room temperature, place the bottom layer on a plate or cake stand. Frost, then add the top layer and frost again. Top with the remaining chopped pecans.

Homemade Dog Treats (Tango's Treats)

Ingredients

1 ¼ cups grated carrots

1 ¼ cups quick-cooking oats

1 cup grated apple

½ cup natural peanut butter

2 eggs

Directions

Preheat the oven to 350 degrees F (175 degrees C). Line 2 baking sheets with parchment paper.

Mix carrots, oats, and apple together in a large bowl. Whisk peanut butter and eggs until thoroughly combined in a second bowl. Pour into the oat mixture and stir until thoroughly combined. Drop 1 1/2 tablespoonfuls of batter onto the prepared baking sheets. Flatten each treat with your hands until they are 1/2-inch thick.

Bake in the preheated oven until treats are firm to the touch and begin to brown on the bottom, 15 to 20 minutes. Allow to cool a few minutes on the baking sheets before removing to a wire rack to cool completely.

Nutrition Facts

Per Serving: 72 calories; protein 3g; carbohydrates 6.3g; fat 4.2g; cholesterol 18.6mg; sodium 29mg.

Pumpkin-Apple Dog Treats

Ingredients

4 cups rolled oats, or as needed

1 medium apple, cored and grated

1 egg

1 cup canned pumpkin

¼ cup rolled oats

Directions

Preheat the oven to 400 degrees F (200 degrees C). Line a baking sheet with parchment paper.

Place 4 cups oatmeal in the bowl of a food processor; pulse until finely ground. Transfer to a mixing bowl.

Stir in grated apple. Mix in canned pumpkin and egg until well combined; mixture will be thick and slightly sticky.

Roll dough on a surface sprinkled with remaining 1/4 cup oats to a 1/2-inch thickness. Cut shapes with a cookie cutter and transfer to the prepared baking sheet.

Bake in the preheated oven until crisp and golden, 12 to 15 minutes. Remove to a wire rack to cool completely.

Nutrition Facts

Per Serving: 64 calories; protein 2.3g; carbohydrates 11.3g; fat 1.2g; cholesterol 7.8mg; sodium 28.4mg.

Conclusion

While surgery that removes or vaporizes the affected area of the brain is the only procedure considered to "cure" epilepsy, it is not always an option – and not always curative. The good news is that other treatments can control most patients' symptoms enough, so they may live normal lives. Patients and loved ones who familiarize themselves with the recognition of epileptic symptoms have a better chance of accurate diagnosis and successful treatment.

Having a precise idea of an individual's epileptic symptoms help ensure that all needs are met. 70% of people with epilepsy achieve remission, and half of those with posttraumatic epilepsy (PTE) achieve remission within the first 15 years.42 Proper diagnosis and treatment is vital in improving management of the condition.

Printed in Great Britain
by Amazon

18011887R00058